VISION REVIVAL

Ginger Powder's Role in Glaucoma and Cataract Condition

JAY ABBAS

Copyright © 2024 by Jay Abbas

All rights reserved. No part of this publication may be reproduced, distributed, or transmitted in any form or by any means, including photocopying, recording, or other electronic or mechanical methods, without the prior written permission of the publisher, except in the case of brief quotations embodied in critical reviews and certain other noncommercial uses permitted by copyright law.

Table of contents

Introduction..3
Chapter 1: The Marvel of Sight: An Introduction to Your Eyes.. 6
Chapter 2: Guardians of Vision: Understanding Eye Care and Maintenance................................. 8
Chapter 3: Glaucoma and Cataracts................. 12
Chapter 4: The Science Behind Ginger's Power.. 17
Chapter 5: The Science Behind Ginger's Eye-Healing Powers..21
Chapter 6: Methodology for Preparing and Applying Ginger to the Eyes.............................25

Introduction

Greetings from the world of herbal knowledge, where the subtle essence of eye care blends with the restorative power of the environment. With much pleasure, I will unravel the complex world of "VISION REVIVAL: Ginger Powder's Role in Glaucoma and Cataract Condition."

Ginger powder is a powerful friend in the fight to preserve eye health when it comes to holistic health. Originating from the rhizome of Zingiber officinale, this fragrant spice has shown extraordinary effects on glaucoma and cataract disorders, in addition to its culinary benefits.

Because of its many benefits, including its anti-inflammatory and antioxidant qualities, ginger is a highly effective natural treatment for eye conditions. The complex interactions among the powerful ingredients in ginger powder may be helpful in reducing inflammation, which is a major cause of glaucoma and cataract development.

Ginger's medicinal potential has been recognized by traditional medicine for centuries, and current research is still revealing more and more of its many advantages. This herbal hero aims to promote a comprehensive approach to eye care in addition to treating symptoms.

Join me on this incredible ride as we examine the deep effects of ginger powder, examining its intricate molecular makeup and the empirical information that has been related down through the ages. "VISION REVIVAL" calls us to appreciate the harmony of the natural world and nourish our eyes with ageless knowledge encased in the golden hue of ginger powder.

Chapter 1: The Marvel of Sight: An Introduction to Your Eyes

The eyes, often referred to as the windows to the soul, are extraordinary sensory organs that grant us the deep ability to perceive and interpret the world around us.

The complex structure of the eye forms the basis of this visual symphony. Imagine your cornea, the clear front portion that lets light in while serving as a shield. The retina, a layer of light-sensitive tissue similar to film in a camera, is the target of light focused by the crystalline lens beyond it. When this light is absorbed by the retina, it is converted into electrical impulses that go down the optic nerve to the brain, where they are processed further.

As we go deeper into the details, take into consideration the iris, the colored part that manages the pupil's size and the quantity of light that enters the eye. Observe the transparent fluids known as the vitreous and aqueous humor, which support and sculpt the tissues of the eye. Together, these elements work in perfect harmony to provide a symphony of functions that facilitate the transformation of light into the vibrant visuals that fill our senses.

But sight is more amazing than just anatomy. Your eyes are dynamic sensors that sense depth, motion, and detail in addition to light's color and intensity. The remarkable intricacy of the ocular system is demonstrated by this complicated dance of visual stimuli.

Chapter 2: Guardians of Vision: Understanding Eye Care and Maintenance

Taking good care of your eyes is like taking care of your vision guardians when it comes to ocular well-being. Entrust the windows to your soul to the care of an expert herbalist. Together, we will explore holistic concepts that go beyond simple maintenance.

The foundation of proper eye care is an understanding of the delicate balance required for the greatest potential vision. The value of routine eye exams should not be overlooked. They act as watchful checks to spot any problems before they materialize. Experts in eye care provide these examinations, which turn into invaluable partners in preserving the health of your eyesight.

Beyond medical evaluations, lifestyle decisions are critical to preserving the guardianship of your eyes. A nutrient-rich diet, enough sleep, and proper hydration all support the general health of your eyes. Think of the eyes as a garden; they flourish when provided with the proper balance of antioxidants, vitamins, and minerals. Eat a variety of vibrant, nutrient defense meals like berries, leafy greens, and omega-3 fatty acids, to strengthen the resilience of your eye garden.

Within the herbal community, certain plant friends become powerful advocates for eye health. The antioxidant-rich bilberry and the calming chamomile are just two of the many herbs found in nature that might help keep your vision vibrant.

- Including these herbs in your daily routine can be a harmonious way to enhance traditional methods of eye care

Consider the impact of environmental factors on the guardianship of your vision. Shield your eyes from excessive sun exposure by donning UV-protective eyewear, a simple yet effective measure to prevent damage from harmful rays.

Conscious attempts to lessen eye strain are essential as the digital age has brought new issues for eye care. To strengthen and relax the ocular muscles, embrace techniques like palming, eye exercises, and blinking exercises. Develop practices that support your general health, understanding that the condition of your eyes has a direct impact on your overall health.

To put it simply, the guardians of eyesight need a comprehensive approach to upkeep and care. Through the integration of clinical vigilance, conscious lifestyle choices, herbal support, and environmental awareness, you strengthen your eyes' resistance to damage.

Chapter 3: Glaucoma and Cataracts

When it comes to eye health, glaucoma and cataracts are two different eye conditions, each with subtle differences. Together, we will explore these eye disorders, highlighting their traits, their causes, and the use of herbal wisdom for their treatment.

Glaucoma

Glaucoma, a complex and progressive eye condition, poses a significant challenge to eye health. let's see the subtleties of glaucoma, including its signs and symptoms, possible causes, and herbal therapeutic options.

Nature of Glaucoma:

Damage to the optic nerve, which is frequently accompanied by an increase in intraocular pressure (IOP), is the hallmark of glaucoma. If treatment is not received, this impairment can lead to permanent blindness as well as a progressive loss of peripheral vision. Glaucoma is known as the "silent thief of sight" because it frequently shows no symptoms in the early stages, leaving affected persons unaware of its presence until substantial vision loss occurs.

Potential Causes and Risk Factors: The specific cause of glaucoma might vary, while high intraocular pressure is a major causing factor. Its development is influenced by age, genetics, and certain medical problems. Its advancement may also be aided by reduced blood supply to the optic nerve and a weakened ability of the nerve to absorb nutrients.

Cataract

The common age-related eye problem known as cataracts causes the natural lens of the eye to fog, impairing vision. Let's discuss the intricacies of cataracts, including their causes, nature, and potential management strategies using herbal treatments.

Nature of Cataracts:

Proteins in the lens of the eye gradually break down and clump together, resulting in cloudiness known as cataracts. When light is obstructed by this clouding, eyesight becomes blurry and in severe cases, is significantly impaired. Although they are frequently linked to age, cataracts can also occur as a result of smoking, diabetes, extended UV exposure, and certain drugs.

Potential Causes and Risk Factors: While age is a primary risk factor, other contributors to cataract formation include:

1. **UV Radiation:** Prolonged exposure to ultraviolet (UV) radiation without adequate care can increase the risk of cataracts.

2. **Smoking:** Tobacco smoke introduces oxidative stress to the eyes, potentially accelerating the development of cataracts.

3. **Medical Conditions:** Diabetes and other medical conditions that impact metabolic processes have a great effect on cataract formation.

Holistic Approach to Glaucoma and Cataracts

A comprehensive approach is required for the holistic care of glaucoma and cataracts, which includes lifestyle changes, traditional therapies (such as surgery in more severe instances), and alternative herbal methods. A holistic approach must include controlling underlying medical issues, preserving a diet high in nutrients, and shielding the eyes from UV light.

Chapter 4: The Science Behind Ginger's Power

Unlocking the potent healing potential of ginger involves deepen into the complex science that underlies its remarkable powers. Let's see the biochemistry of ginger, unraveling the scientific tapestry that makes this humble root a powerhouse of health benefits.

Active Compounds in Ginger:

Ginger (Zingiber officinale) harbors a rich reservoir of bioactive compounds that contribute to its therapeutic properties. One such group is gingerols, known for their anti-inflammatory and antioxidant effects. These compounds are the primary reason behind ginger's distinct taste and aroma.

Anti-Inflammatory Properties:

Inflammation is a natural response of the body to injury or infection, but chronic inflammation is associated with various health issues. Gingerols, particularly 6-gingerol, exhibit potent anti-inflammatory effects by inhibiting inflammatory pathways at the molecular level. This makes ginger a valuable ally in managing conditions linked to inflammation, from arthritis to gastrointestinal discomfort.

Antioxidant Defense:

Ginger's antioxidant prowess is attributed to its ability to neutralize free radicals, unstable molecules that can damage cells and contribute to various chronic diseases. The antioxidant compounds in ginger, including gingerols, offer cellular protection by scavenging free radicals, thereby aiding in the prevention of oxidative stress.

Modulating Cellular Responses:

Beyond its direct antioxidant and anti-inflammatory actions, ginger influences cellular signaling pathways. Studies suggest that gingerols may modulate certain genes and proteins involved in inflammatory responses, exerting a regulatory effect on the body's intricate cellular machinery.

Gastrointestinal Benefits:

Ginger has a long history of use in alleviating digestive discomfort. Its ability to stimulate saliva production and suppress gastric contractions may contribute to its anti-nausea and anti-vomiting effects. Additionally, ginger has been explored for its potential in promoting gastrointestinal motility and relieving indigestion.

Cardiovascular Support:

Research indicates that ginger may contribute to cardiovascular health by positively influencing factors such as blood pressure and cholesterol levels. Its anti-inflammatory and antioxidant properties play a role in maintaining the integrity of blood vessels and supporting overall heart health.

Culinary and Medicinal Harmony:
Ginger's versatility extends beyond its medicinal attributes. Its use in culinary creations not only enhances flavor but also introduces its therapeutic compounds into daily diets. From teas and infusions to savory dishes and desserts, ginger seamlessly integrates into a variety of preparations, offering both gastronomic delight and health benefits.

Chapter 5: The Science Behind Ginger's Eye-Healing Powers

Rhizomes of the Zingiber officinale plant, ginger are rich in bioactive components that support the health of the eyes, which is one of its many unique medicinal properties.

Gingerols Anti-Inflammatory Ballet:

One of the most important components of ginger is gingerol, a bioactive compound with potent anti-inflammatory properties. Many conditions affecting the eyes, such as conjunctivitis and dry eyes, are characterized by inflammation. Research has shown that gingerol can block inflammatory pathways, which can provide relief for those who are experiencing pain and redness. Gingerol is an all-natural ally for relieving inflamed eyes since it regulates inflammatory reactions.

Zingerone's Antioxidant Shield:

Another important component in ginger's healing ability is zingerone, a phenolic compound with robust antioxidant capabilities. The eyes immensely benefit from zingerone's capacity to neutralize free radicals since they are particularly vulnerable to oxidative stress. Degenerative eye disorders such as age-related macular degeneration are associated with oxidative stress. Zingerone provides a shielding effect by acting as an antioxidant, reducing cellular damage that may cause visual impairment.

Nourishing Nutrients for Optimal Vision:

Apart from gingerol and zingerone, ginger contains an array of essential nutrients that are vital for maintaining optimal eye health. Vitamins such as vitamin C and vitamin A, present in ginger, contribute to the nourishment of ocular tissues. These nutrients play a vital role in preventing conditions like night blindness and supporting overall visual acuity.

Balancing Blood Circulation to the Eyes:

The health of our eyes depends critically on effective blood circulation. Because of the vasodilatory actions of ginger, blood flow is improved and essential nutrients are delivered to the eyes in large quantities. Increased circulation can help avoid diseases like glaucoma that are brought on by inadequate blood flow.

Synergistic Effects in Eye Care:

The synergistic benefits of ginger's numerous components are what make its healing properties so beautiful. Zingerone, gingerol, and the abundance of nutrients come together to form a harmonic combination that not only treats particular eye disorders but also supports the health of the visual system as a whole. Because of its synergistic action, ginger stands out as a comprehensive treatment for keeping eyes bright and healthy.

Chapter 6: Methodology for Preparing and Applying Ginger to the Eyes

1. Start by acquiring fresh ginger. Ensure it's clean and free from any dirt or impurities.

2. Thoroughly wash the ginger under running water to remove any remaining soil or debris.

3. Using a clean crusher or a mortar and pestle, carefully squash the washed ginger until you extract the water content. This process may involve gentle crushing to release the oil from the ginger.

4. Choose a clean container to collect the extracted ginger oil. This container should be free from any

contaminants to maintain the purity of the oil.

5. For a more comfortable application and to reduce potential irritation, dilute the ginger oil with a small amount of hot water. Stir the mixture well to ensure proper blending.

6. Once you've achieved the desired dilution, transfer the ginger oil mixture into a sterile eyedrop container. This container should be thoroughly cleaned and sanitized to prevent any bacterial contamination.

7. Apply the diluted ginger oil to your eyes before bedtime. Use the provided eyedropper for precise and controlled application.

8. Consistently apply the mixture every night for a duration of two weeks to observe potential benefits.

Printed in Great Britain
by Amazon